Natural Antibiotics
&
Antiviral Remedies

Background on Natural Remedies and 50 Homemade Recipes

Table of Contents

Introduction

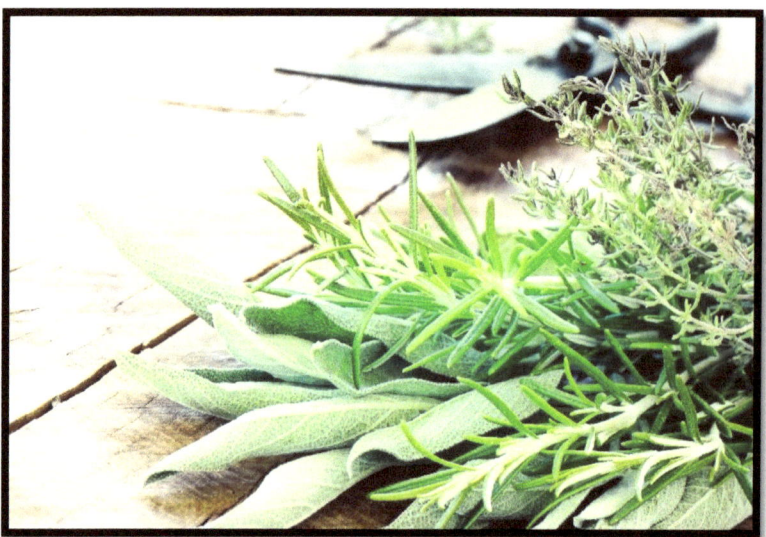

For many people, the first thing they do when they detect a hint of illness is call the family doctor. But what if you could treat common illnesses without even having to leave your house? Rather than pumping your family full of prescription drugs that can have unpleasant, or even dangerous side effects, why not turn to a more natural course of treatment – antibiotic and antiviral herbs.

Natural remedies for common illnesses have existed for thousands of years, but many people have forgotten about them. In this book you will learn the basics about these remedies including their benefits and how to use them. You will receive a list of the top 10 antiviral and antibacterial herbs as well as a collection of homemade recipes to make your own antiviral and antibiotic remedies at home. Never again will you have to subject your family to the effects of ineffective antibiotic medications.

Benefits of Natural Remedies

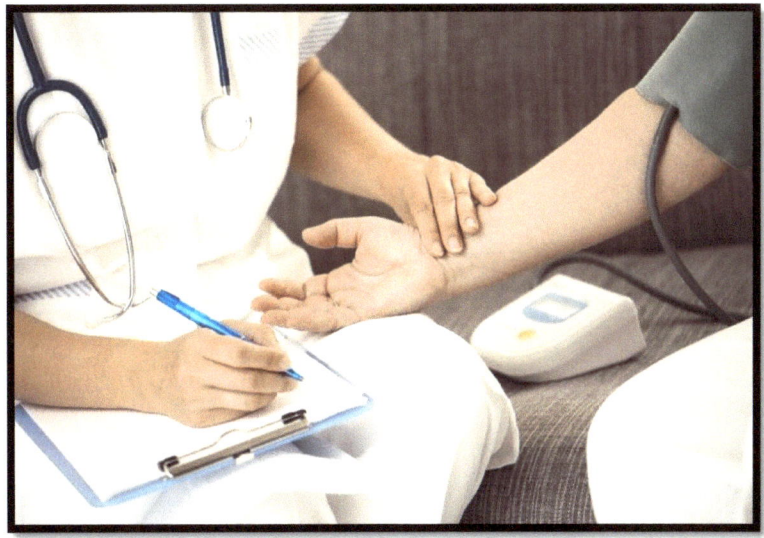

When penicillin was first discovered, it was thought to be a miracle drug – all of a sudden, bacterial infections caused by staphylococci and streptococci were no longer a threat. Over the years, however, misuse and over-prescription of antibiotics has led to an increase in antibiotic resistance. Whereas antibiotic production in 1954 totaled about 2 million pounds, that number leapt to more than 54 million pounds by the year 2000. In fact, it is estimated that more than ¾ of the antibiotics prescribed by doctors today are entirely unnecessary. Antibiotic medications that were once incredibly effective now fail to put even a dent in the effects of common bacterial diseases. If antibiotic prescriptions are no longer effect, what options are left?

Perhaps the best course of action is not to pursue more effective prescription antibiotics but to return to a more natural course of treatment – antibiotic and antiviral herbs. There are a vast number of herbs, spices, and plants that have been used in traditional medicine for centuries to treat common bacterial infections like cold and flu. The best part about these remedies is that they are all-natural – they do not cause the side effects that have been linked to antibiotic prescriptions and they are even effective against bacteria that no longer respond to antibiotic drugs. In the following pages you will receive an overview of some of the top antibacterial and antiviral herbs and plants that can be used as a natural treatment for bacterial infections.

Herbs with Antibiotic/Antiviral Properties

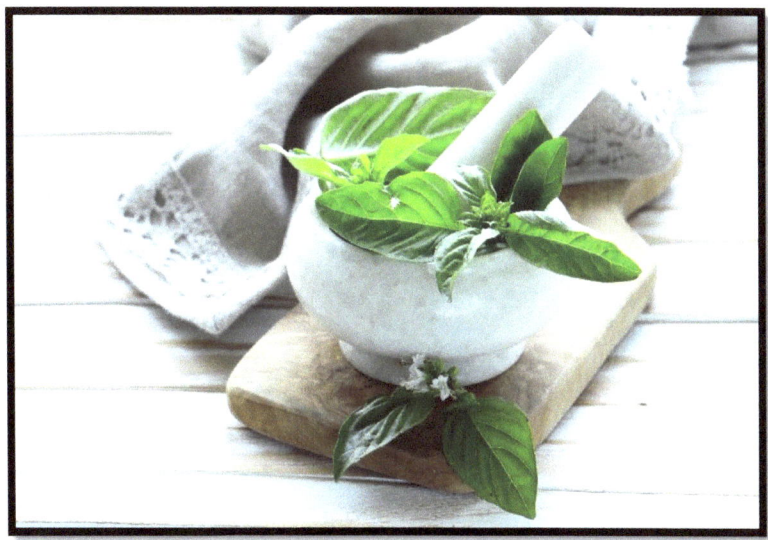

As you learned in the previous sections, prescription antibiotics are misused and over-prescribed. In many cases, they also cause unpleasant side effects that leave you wondering whether it is worth taking them at all. Fortunately, there is a simple and all-natural alternative – herbal antibiotics and antivirals. In this section you will receive an overview of the top 10 antibiotic and antiviral herbs that will be used in the next section for homemade antibiotic and antiviral recipes.

Top 10 Antibiotic Herbs

Basil – Basil (*Ocimum basilicum*) is a very common herb that provides a number of powerful antibiotic benefits. This herb has been used to treat stomach spasms, gas, and fluid retention as well as intestinal worms and head colds – it can also be used as an appetite stimulant. When applied topically, basil can help to promote blood circulation and it can also relieve inflammation and pain due to snake or insect bites.

Calendula – The flowers of the calendula (*Calendula officinalis*) plant are known for their antibiotic benefits. Calendula is widely used as an herbal treatment for wounds, though it can also be taken internally to treat sore throat, stomach ulcers, and menstrual cramps. This herb is also popular as a fever-reducer.

Cinnamon – Cinnamon (*Cinnamomum verum*) is derived from the bark of the cinnamon tree and it is used for both culinary and medicinal applications. This spice is often added to tea to warm the body and aid in digestion but its essential oil can be applied topically to increase blood flow. The antibiotic benefits of cinnamon have been shown to help treat upset stomach, gas, diarrhea, cramps, cold and flu.

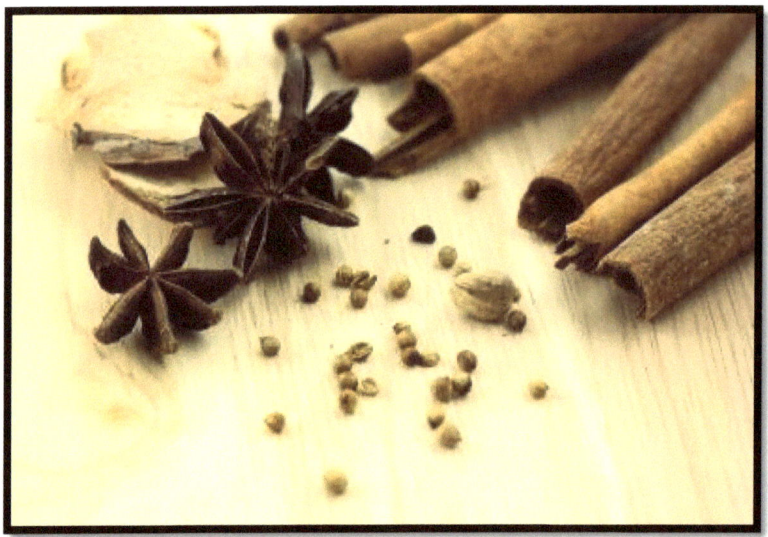

Clove – The leaves, stems and buds of the clove plant (*Syzgium aromaticum*) provide powerful antibacterial properties. When applied topically, clove acts as an analgesic and, when taken internally, it is useful in killing bad bacteria. Clove has been shown to be effective as a treatment for nausea, diarrhea, vomiting and stomach upset.

Echinacea – The power of Echinacea (*Achinacea angustifolia*) lies in its ability to prevent or reduce the duration of cold and flu. This herb has also been used to treat yeast infections, urinary tract infections, strep throat, and septicemia. When applied to the skin, Echinacea is a good treatment for abscesses, boils, wounds, burns, and bee stings as well as skin conditions like eczema and psoriasis.

Garlic – Not only is garlic (*Allium sativum*) a flavorful culinary ingredient, but it is also has powerful antibacterial benefits as well. Garlic is actually more effective against certain types of bacteria than penicillin and other penicillin antibiotics. The most important benefit of garlic that while it kills pathogenic bacteria, it is gentle on gut flora. Garlic can be used to treat cough, headache, fever, asthma and bronchitis as well as various skin conditions.

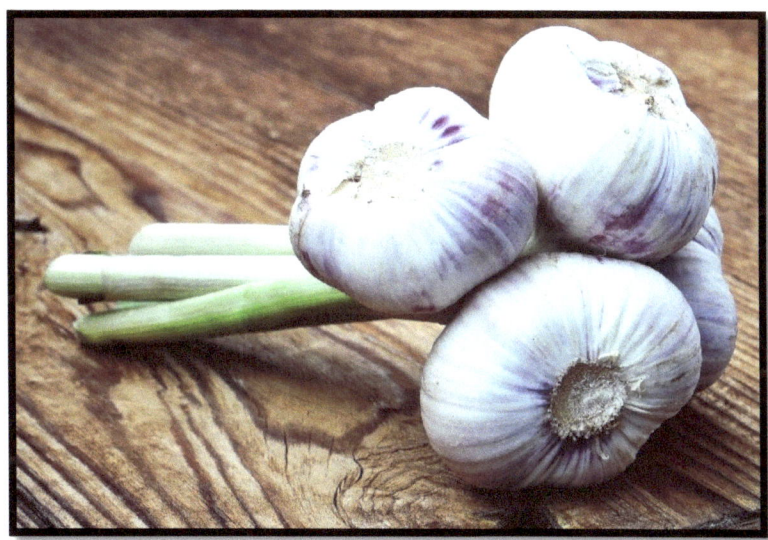

Myrrh – Myrrh is the aromatic resin of the *Commihpora myrrha* tree and it has been used for centuries in various herbal remedies. In addition to its antibacterial properties, myrrh is also used as a treatment for cold, cough, asthma, congestion, and ulcers.

When applied topically, myrrh can be used to treat mouth soreness and swelling, gum inflammation, canker sores, and chapped lips.

Oregon Grape – The root of the Oregon grape plant (*Mahonia aquifolium*) is a powerful antibacterial agent that has been used to treat stomach upset, stomach ulcers, internal bacterial infections, and various other gastrointestinal diseases. When applied topically, Oregon grape root can be used as a disinfectant and as a treatment for psoriasis and various other skin conditions.

Sage – A fragrant perennial herb, sage (*Salvia officinalis*) is known for its antibacterial properties and other medicinal benefits. This herb has been used as a treatment for various digestive problems including gas, stomach pain, diarrhea, bloating and heartburn – it can also help with depression and memory loss. When applied, topically, sage can help to treat cold sores, gum disease, and sore throat.

Thyme – Thyme (*Thymus vulgaris)* is a flowering herb that is used for both culinary and medicinal applications. The antibacterial benefits of this herb are primarily beneficial in treating respiratory conditions such as sore throat, cough, and bronchitis but thyme can also be used to treat arthritis, stomach pain, gas, and parasitic infections.

Top 10 Antiviral Herbs

Astragalus Root – Astragalus root (*Astragalus membranaceus*) is a type of legume that provides antiviral benefits by boosting the immune system. This herb is primarily beneficial as a precautionary measure, helping to prevent flu and cold. Astragalus root can also be used to treat arthritis, asthma, and upper respiratory infections.

Cranberry – Though it is not technically an herb, cranberry (*Vaccinium macrocarpon*) is still a powerful natural antiviral. This fruit is particularly beneficial as a treatment against urinary tract infections and for bladder disease. Cranberry has also been used to relieve the symptoms of type 2 diabetes, chronic fatigue syndrome, scurvy, and certain cancers.

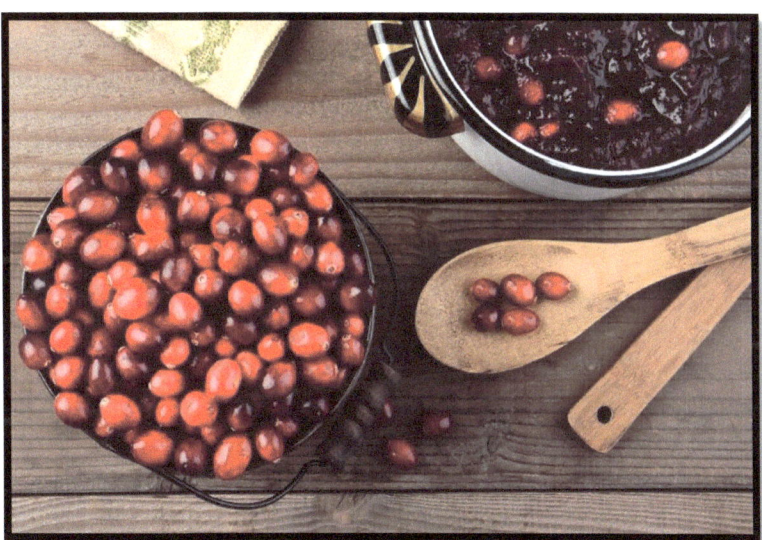

Elderberry – Not only is the common black elderberry (*Sambucas nigra*) a food source, but it is also a powerful antiviral. This herb has been used for centuries in a variety of natural remedies for flue, HIV, herpes, and other viral diseases. In several studies, patients taking elderberry were seen to have a significant reduction in flu symptoms after just two days.

Ginger – Ginger (*Zingiber officinale*) is known for both its antiviral and antibacterial properties. This herb contains a number of powerful compounds such as gingerols, zingerone, and shogaol which are the active ingredients that make ginger so medicinally useful. Ginger has been used to prevent and decrease the severity of colds and as a treatment for nausea, stomach ache, gas, and diarrhea.

Lemon Balm – The efficacy of lemon balm (*Melissa officinalis*) comes from the volatile oil which provides strong antiviral benefits. Lemon balm has been used to treat stomach upset as well as colic, gas, bloating, and menstrual cramps. It can also be applied topically as a treatment for cold sores.

Licorice – The root of the licorice plant (*Glycyrrhiza glabra*) is known for its antiviral properties, especially its efficacy against the SARS virus. Not only is licorice a powerful antiviral, but it is non-toxic to virus-infected cells – it only targets the virus itself. Licorice can be used as a treatment for HIV, hepatitis, gastric ulcers, and various other viruses.

Mullein – Mullein (*Verbascum thapsus*) is an herb that is known for its gentle antiviral antibacterial properties – this makes it particularly popular as an herbal remedy for children. This herb has been used to treat ear infections as well as headache, fever, flue, cold, and pneumonia. Mullein is particularly effective in combination with garlic.

Olive Leaf – The leaves of the olive tree (*Olea europea*) are known for their healing properties, especially in relation to cardiovascular health. The healing power of olive leaves comes from a bitter compound called oleuropein which has strong antiviral properties. Olive leaf has been effective as a treatment for influenza, herpes, polio, and a variety of viral skin infections.

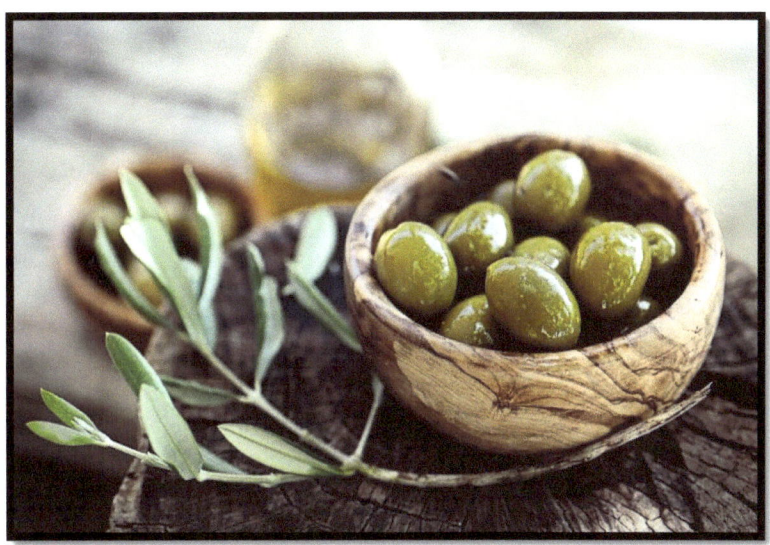

Oregano – Oregano (*Origanum vulgare*) is a fragrant herb that has been used for centuries in natural herbal remedies for various viral conditions. This herb is an effective treatment for respiratory tract conditions as well as gastrointestinal disorders and intestinal parasites. Oregano can be used to treat various skin conditions as well, including acne, warts, rosacea, ringworm, and psoriasis.

St. John's Wort – Though St. John's Wort (*Hypericum perforatum*) is primarily known as an herbal treatment for depression, it also has strong antiviral benefits. This herb has been used to speed wound healing and to ease pain associated with various conditions. In regard to its antiviral properties, St. John's Wort has been used to treat influenza, herpes, HIV, and other viral conditions.

Recipes for Homemade Antibiotic and Antiviral Remedies

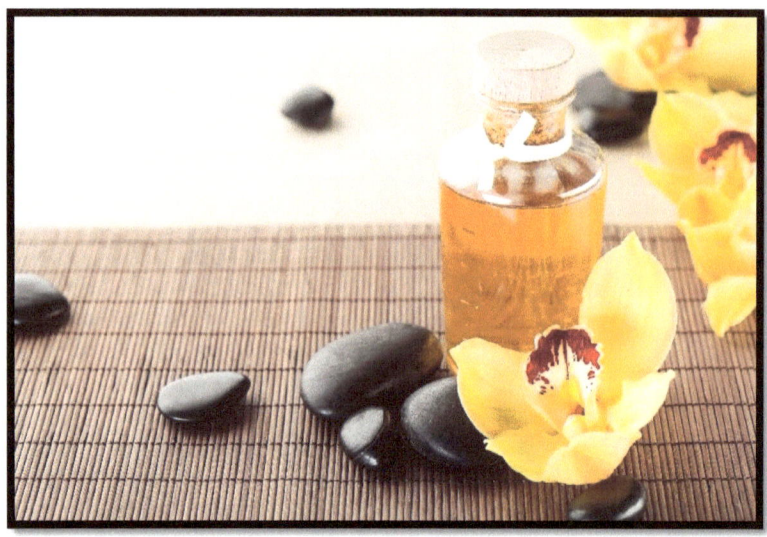

When it comes to making your own natural antibiotic remedies at home, there are a variety of different forms they can take. In this book you will find a collection of recipes for various applications including skin conditions, internal infections, general maladies, and more. Below you will find a list of the categories into which these recipes will be divided.

Recipes Included in this Book:

Topical Salves and Ointments

Teas, Tinctures and Infusions

Other Antibiotic Recipes

Topical Salves and Ointments

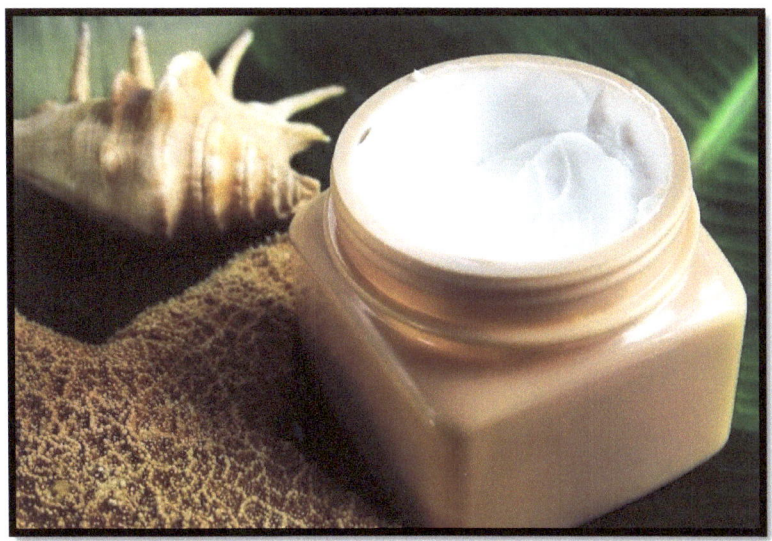

<u>Recipes Included in this Section</u>:

Easy Antibiotic Ointment

Sunburn Soothing Cream

Eczema Salve with Calendula

Stimulating Cinnamon Salve

Soothing Diaper Rash Cream

Peppermint Antibiotic Ointment

Ginger Salve for Burns

Arthritis-Soothing Myrrh Salve

Psoriasis Ointment with Oregon Grape

Basil Cream for Insect Bites

Easy Antibiotic Ointment

This easy antibiotic ointment is the perfect all-purpose antibiotic to have on hand for cuts, scrapes, and burns. Feel free to customize the scent of this ointment by using your favorite essential oils.

Ingredients:

2 ounces sweet almond oil

2 ounces jojoba oil

2 tablespoons grated beeswax

10 drops tea tree oil

5 drops lime essential oil

5 drops Echinacea essential oil

Instructions:

1. Combine the sweet almond oil, jojoba oil and beeswax in a double boiler over low heat.
2. Once the beeswax has melted, stir the ingredients well to combine.
3. Remove from heat and cool to room temperature.
4. Stir in the essential oils until thoroughly combined.
5. Pour the mixture into a metal tin or glass jar and cover with the lid.
6. Store the ointment in a cool, dry area.
7. Apply the ointment to clean skin as a treatment for wounds, burns, and cuts.

Sunburn Soothing Cream

This sunburn soothing cream is made with natural ingredients that will both soothe and heal your skin. Lavender not only has antibacterial properties, but will also help to prevent itching while coconut oil and shea butter moisturize your skin.

Ingredients:

3 tablespoons dried lavender, crushed

¼ cup water

2 tablespoons shea butter

2 tablespoons coconut oil

1 tablespoon beeswax

1 tablespoon sweet almond oil

4 drops tea tree essential oil

Small glass jar

Instructions:

1. Stir together the lavender and water in a small saucepan.
2. Bring the mixture to a simmer over medium-low heat – simmer for 12 to 15 minutes.
3. Remove from heat and strain the mixture into a small bowl, discarding the solids.
4. Melt the beeswax, shea butter, sweet almond oil, and coconut oil in a double boiler over low heat.
5. Spoon 2 tablespoons of the reserved liquid along with the tea tree essential oil into the double boiler and stir well.
6. Pour the mixture into a small glass jar and cover tightly with the lid.
7. Spread the cream on clean, dry skin to relieve the itching and irritation of sunburn.

Eczema Salve with Calendula

Eczema is a skin condition in which the skin becomes inflamed and irritated. This salve made with calendula flowers is a natural, herbal remedy for eczema that soothes irritated skin and promotes healing.

Ingredients:

1/3 cup extra-virgin olive oil

¼ cup dried calendula flowers, crushed

1 tablespoon grated beeswax

Small glass jar with lid

Water, as needed

Instructions:

1. Fill a deep skillet with several inches of water and bring it to a slow boil.
2. Pour the calendula into a glass jar then add the olive oil.
3. Stir gently so the calendula is saturated.
4. Place the jar in the boiling water – if needed, remove some water from the skillet to ensure that none gets into the jar.
5. Simmer the jar in warm water over low heat for 4 to 5 hours.
6. Remove the skillet from heat and set the jar aside until it is cool enough to handle.
7. Pour the contents of the jar through a mesh strainer and squeeze as much oil as you can from the calendula.
8. Return the liquid to the jar and pour in the grated beeswax.
9. Place the jar back in the skillet for a few minutes until the beeswax is melted – stir to incorporate.
10. Remove the jar from the water and cool to room temperature, stirring occasionally.
11. Use the salve to relieve the itching, inflammation, and irritation of eczema.
12. Store in a cool, dry location with the lid tightly secured.

Stimulating Cinnamon Salve

Not only does cinnamon provide antibacterial benefits, but it has also been shown to help stimulate blood flow. Use this salve to moisturize and revitalize dry or sun-damaged skin. Feel free to add other essential oils to change the fragrance.

Ingredients:

¼ cup sweet almond oil

¼ cup jojoba oil

¼ cup extra-virgin olive oil

2 tablespoons coconut oil

1 tablespoon grated beeswax

½ cup rose water

¼ teaspoon vitamin E oil

8 drops cinnamon essential oil

Instructions:

1. Combine the sweet almond oil, jojoba oil, olive oil and coconut oil in a double boiler over low heat.
2. Once the oils star to melt, stir in the beeswax and whisk well until it has completely dissolved.
3. In a mixing bowl, whisk together the rose water, vitamin E oil, and cinnamon essential oil.
4. While whisking, slowly pour the melted oils into the rose water mixture.
5. Whisk until the mixture is smooth and creamy.
6. Transfer the mixture to a small jar or metal tin and cover with the lid.
7. Store in the cool, dry place and use as you would any other moisturizer or salve.

Soothing Diaper Rash Cream

Diaper rash can be both irritating and painful for children in addition to being difficult to treat, in some cases. This soothing diaper rash cream is made with natural antibiotic herbs to soothe and heal the rash naturally and effectively.

Ingredients:

3 tablespoons dried calendula, crushed

¼ cup water

2 tablespoons shea butter

1 ½ tablespoons coconut oil

1 ½ tablespoons beeswax

1 tablespoon olive oil

Small glass jar

Instructions:

1. Stir together the calendula and water in a small saucepan.
2. Bring the mixture to a simmer over medium-low heat – simmer for 12 to 15 minutes.
3. Remove from heat and strain the mixture into a small bowl, discarding the solids.
4. Melt the beeswax, shea butter, olive oil, and coconut oil in a double boiler over low heat.
5. Spoon 2 tablespoons of the reserved liquid into the double boiler and stir well.
6. Pour the mixture into a small glass jar and cover tightly with the lid.
7. Spread the cream on clean, dry skin to relieve the symptoms of diaper rash.

Peppermint Antibiotic Ointment

This antibiotic ointment has the added power of peppermint essential oil which has been shown to provide antibacterial, antiseptic, and anti-inflammatory benefits. More importantly, it smells great!

Ingredients:

2 ounces sweet almond oil

2 ounces jojoba oil

2 tablespoons grated beeswax

10 drops tea tree oil

6 drops peppermint essential oil

3 drops eucalyptus essential oil

Instructions:

1. Combine the sweet almond oil, jojoba oil and beeswax in a double boiler over low heat.
2. Once the beeswax has melted, stir the ingredients well to combine.
3. Remove from heat and cool to room temperature.
4. Stir in the essential oils until thoroughly combined.
5. Pour the mixture into a metal tin or glass jar and cover with the lid.
6. Store the ointment in a cool, dry area.
7. Apply the ointment to clean skin as a treatment for wounds, burns, and cuts.

Ginger Salve for Burns

Ginger is a powerful antibacterial herb that can also be used topically to treat burns. This ginger salve is just what you need to soothe and heal all kinds of burns from sunburn to 1st and 2nd-degree burns.

Ingredients:

¼ cup sweet almond oil

¼ cup extra-virgin olive oil

3 tablespoons jojoba oil

2 tablespoons coconut oil

1 tablespoon grated beeswax

½ cup rose water

¼ teaspoon vitamin E oil

8 drops ginger essential oil

Instructions:

1. Combine the sweet almond oil, jojoba oil, olive oil and coconut oil in a double boiler over low heat.
2. Once the oils star to melt, stir in the beeswax and whisk well until it has completely dissolved.
3. In a mixing bowl, whisk together the rose water, vitamin E oil, and ginger essential oil.
4. While whisking, slowly pour the melted oils into the rose water mixture.
5. Whisk until the mixture is smooth and creamy.
6. Transfer the mixture to a small jar or metal tin and cover with the lid.
7. Store in the cool, dry place and use as you would any other moisturizer or salve.

Arthritis-Soothing Salve with Thyme and Myrrh

This soothing salve is made with two powerful antibiotic and anti-inflammatory herbs – thyme and myrrh. Spread this salve on sore joints and ligaments and use it to relieve the pain and inflammation associated with arthritis.

Ingredients:

¾ cup extra-virgin olive oil

½ cup dried thyme, crushed

2 ½ tablespoons grated beeswax

8 drops myrrh essential oil

Small glass jar with lid

Water, as needed

Instructions:

1. Fill a deep skillet with several inches of water and bring it to a slow boil.
2. Pour the dried thyme into a glass jar then add the olive oil.
3. Stir gently so the thyme is saturated.
4. Place the jar in the boiling water – if needed, remove some water from the skillet to ensure that none gets into the jar.
5. Simmer the jar in warm water over low heat for 4 to 5 hours.
6. Remove the skillet from heat and set the jar aside until it is cool enough to handle.
7. Pour the contents of the jar through a mesh strainer and squeeze as much oil as you can from the thyme.
8. Return the liquid to the jar and pour in the grated beeswax.
9. Place the jar back in the skillet for a few minutes until the beeswax is melted – stir to incorporate then stir in the myrrh essential oil.
10. Remove the jar from the water and cool to room temperature, stirring occasionally.
11. Store in a cool, dry location with the lid tightly secured.

Psoriasis Ointment with Oregon Grape Root

Psoriasis is a fairly common skin condition that results from a change in the life cycle of skin cells. In cases of psoriasis, cells accumulate rapidly on the surface of the skin which leads to scaly, dry patches of itchy skin. This herbal ointment made with Oregon grape root will help to naturally soothe and heal psoriasis.

Ingredients:

1/3 cup extra-virgin olive oil

¼ cup dried Oregon grape root, crushed

1 ½ tablespoons grated beeswax

Small glass jar with lid

Water, as needed

Instructions:

1. Fill a deep skillet with several inches of water and bring it to a slow boil.
2. Pour the Oregon grape root into a glass jar then add the olive oil.
3. Stir gently so the Oregon grape root is saturated.
4. Place the jar in the boiling water – if needed, remove water from the skillet to ensure that none gets into the jar.
5. Simmer the jar in warm water over low heat for 4 to 5 hours.
6. Remove the skillet from heat and set the jar aside until it is cool enough to handle.
7. Pour the contents of the jar through a mesh strainer and squeeze as much oil as you can from the Oregon grape root.
8. Return the liquid to the jar and pour in the grated beeswax.
9. Place the jar back in the skillet for a few minutes until the beeswax is melted – stir to incorporate.
10. Remove the jar from the water and cool to room temperature, stirring occasionally.
11. Use the salve to relieve the irritation and itching caused by psoriasis.
12. Store in a cool, dry location with the lid tightly secured.

Basil Cream for Insect Bites

This herbal cream is the perfect remedy for insect bites. The antibiotic power of basil helps to heal the bite while the cooling power of arnica flowers reduces inflammation and soothes irritation.

Ingredients:

½ cup coconut oil

½ tablespoon dried arnica flowers, crushed

2 tablespoons grated beeswax

4 drops basil essential oil

1 drop eucalyptus essential oil

Instructions:

1. Melt the coconut oil in a double boiler over low heat.
2. Stir in the dried arnica flowers and simmer the mixture on low heat for at least 12 hours, stirring occasionally.
3. Remove from heat and let the mixture cool for 20 minutes.
4. Strain the mixture through cheesecloth, squeezing as much oil from the arnica flowers as possible.
5. Pour the oil back into the double boiler and stir in the grated beeswax.
6. Warm the mixture until the beeswax is melted and stir to combine.
7. Remove from heat and stir in the essential oils then pour the mixture into a small glass or metal container.
8. Spread the cream on clean, dry skin to relieve itching and inflammation from insect bites.

Teas, Tinctures and Infusions

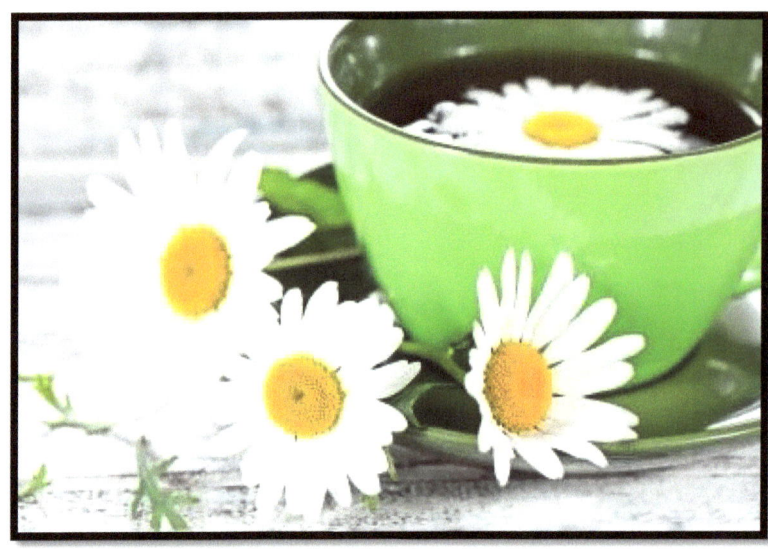

Recipes Included in this Section:

Echinacea Tincture for Cold and Flu

Cinnamon Clove Herbal Tea

Ginger Infusion for Intestinal Bacteria

Fever-Reducing Calendula Tincture

Mint Infusion for Congestion

Lemon Balm Tea for Headache

Cough-Reducing Ginger Tincture

Sage Gargle for Sore Throat

Immune-Boosting Licorice Tincture

Antibiotic Garlic Infusion

Sage Tincture for Sore Throat

Turmeric Tea with Ginger

Echinacea Tincture for Cold and Flu

Echinacea is widely known for preventing and reducing the duration of cold and flu. This Echinacea tincture is easy to make but it does take a little time to prepare, so make it a few weeks before flu season starts so you will have it on hand.

Ingredients:

¼ cup dried Echinacea, crushed

1 ¼ cups high-proof vodka

Glass pint jar

Instructions:

1. Pour the Echinacea into the pint jar.
2. Add the vodka and stir until the herbs are fully saturated.
3. Screw the lid tightly onto the jar and place it in a cool, dark area.
4. Let the jar sit for 2 weeks, shaking it once daily.
5. Strain the mixture through a piece of cheesecloth, squeezing the liquid from the herbs as much as possible.
6. Discard the solids and strain the liquid through a coffee filter.
7. Pour the liquid into small, dark-colored glass bottles.
8. To use, take ½ to 1 teaspoon of the tincture directly by mouth 3 to 4 times daily when you feel cold or flu coming on.

Cinnamon Clove Herbal Tea

Not only can cinnamon boost your memory and alertness, but it can also aid digestion. Both cinnamon and clove are natural antibiotic remedies for various forms of digestive upset.

Ingredients:

1 ½ cups water

1 (3 inch) cinnamon stick

2 whole cloves

Instructions:

1. Pour the water into a small saucepan and add the cinnamon and clove.
2. Bring to a slow boil over medium-low heat.
3. Simmer for 5 minutes over low heat until bubbling.
4. Remove the saucepan from the heat and let steep for 15 minutes.
5. Strain the liquid through a mesh strainer or cheesecloth.
6. Reheat the tea, if needed, and enjoy immediately.

Ginger Infusion for Intestinal Bacteria

Ginger is one of the most powerful natural antibiotics and it can be used to treat a number of bacterial infections. This ginger infusion is a wonderful multi-purpose treatment for intestinal bacteria.

Ingredients:

½ cup fresh minced ginger

¾ cups extra-virgin olive oil

½ cup hot water

Instructions:

1. Place the ginger in a small glass jar and pour in the olive oil.
2. Cover the jar tightly with a lid and place in a sunny area.
3. Let the jar sit for 2 weeks, shaking twice a day to keep the ginger submerged.
4. After 2 weeks, strain the mixture through cheesecloth and discard the ginger.
5. Pour the oil back into the small jar and store in the refrigerator.
6. Add 1 teaspoon of the infusion to ½ cup of hot water and enjoy daily.

Fever-Reducing Calendula Tincture

Not only is calendula a great herb for treating sore throats, but it can also be used to reduce fever. This calendula tincture is one of the easiest ways to reap the benefits of the herb, so be sure to have a jar of it on hand.

Ingredients:

¼ cup dried calendula flowers, crushed

1 ¼ cups high-proof rum

Glass pint jar

Instructions:

1. Pour the calendula flowers into the pint jar.
2. Add the rum and stir until the herbs are fully saturated.
3. Screw the lid tightly onto the jar and place it in a cool, dark area.
4. Let the jar sit for 2 weeks, shaking it once daily.
5. Strain the mixture through a piece of cheesecloth, squeezing the liquid from the herbs as much as possible.
6. Discard the solids and strain the liquid through a coffee filter.
7. Pour the liquid into small, dark-colored glass bottles.
8. To use, take ½ to 1 teaspoon of the tincture directly by mouth or in tea to reduce fever.

Mint Infusion for Congestion

The mint family of herbs is known for providing a wide variety of medicinal benefits. In addition to having a pleasant fragrance and uplifting aroma, mint is also a powerful expectorant. Use this mint infusion to relieve chest or nasal congestion.

Ingredients:

Boiling water

Handful fresh mint leaves

Heat-proof bowl

Towel

Instructions:

1. Bring several inches of water to boil in a small saucepan.
2. Stir in the fresh mint leaves then cover and steep for 15 minutes.
3. Pour the liquid into a heat-proof bowl and set it on the table in front of you.
4. Lean over the bowl and cover your head with a towel to contain the steam.
5. Inhale the vapors deeply for 5 to 10 minutes.

Lemon Balm Tea for Headache

Not only is lemon balm pleasantly fragrant, but it is also a powerful herbal remedy for headaches. This homemade lemon balm tea will have you feeling better in no time – it is especially effective against headaches that are accompanied by nausea.

Ingredients:

1 teaspoon fresh chopped lemon balm

1 cup boiling water

Honey to taste

Instructions:

1. Place the lemon balm in a mug or tea cup.
2. Pour in the boiling water and let steep for several minutes.
3. Sweeten with honey to taste and enjoy immediately.

Cough-Reducing Ginger Tincture

Ginger is a natural expectorant which means it is perfect for helping to reduce cough. Take this ginger tincture directly by mouth or add it to a warm cup of tea to enhance its cough-reducing effects.

Ingredients:

¼ cup fresh grated ginger

1 ¼ cups high-proof vodka

Glass pint jar

Instructions:

1. Pour the ginger into the pint jar.
2. Add the vodka and stir until the herbs are fully saturated.
3. Screw the lid tightly onto the jar and place it in a cool, dark area.
4. Let the jar sit for 2 weeks, shaking it once daily.
5. Strain the mixture through a piece of cheesecloth, squeezing the liquid from the ginger as much as possible.
6. Discard the solids and strain the liquid through a coffee filter.
7. Pour the liquid into small, dark-colored glass bottles.
8. To use, take ½ to 1 teaspoon of the tincture directly by mouth 3 to 4 times daily or add it to a cup of warm tea.

Sage Gargle for Sore Throat

In addition to its other medicinal benefits, sage is widely known for its ability to soothe a sore throat. This recipe will guide you through the process to make homemade sage tea which, with the addition of Epsom salts, can be made into a gargle as well.

Ingredients:

10 fresh sage leaves

8 ounces boiling water

¼ teaspoon Epsom salt

Instructions:

1. Place the sage leaves in a large mug.
2. Pour in 8 ounces of boiling water and let steep for 5 minutes.
3. Strain the mixture, discarding the sage leaves.
4. Divide the tea between two mugs and stir the salt into one mug.
5. Let the sage-salt tea cool slightly then gargle with it to soothe a sore throat.
6. Drink the remaining sage tea to further soothe your throat.

Immune-Boosting Licorice Tincture

Licorice is a powerful antibacterial herb that provides a wide variety of medicinal benefits. Not only can it help to soothe a sore throat and reduce cough, but it can also boost your immune system to help you fight off infection.

Ingredients:

¼ cup dried licorice root

1 ¼ cups high-proof rum

Glass pint jar

Instructions:

1. Pour the licorice root into the pint jar.
2. Add the rum and stir until the herbs are fully saturated.
3. Screw the lid tightly onto the jar and place it in a cool, dark area.
4. Let the jar sit for 2 weeks, shaking it once daily.
5. Strain the mixture through a piece of cheesecloth, squeezing the liquid from the licorice root as much as possible.
6. Discard the solids and strain the liquid through a coffee filter.
7. Pour the liquid into small, dark-colored glass bottles.
8. To use, take ½ to 1 teaspoon of the tincture directly by mouth 3 to 4 times daily when you feel cold or flu coming on.

Antibiotic Garlic Infusion

The main medicinal benefit of garlic is that it is a powerful antibiotic – it is also a great source of antioxidants. This garlic infusion can be used for everything from yeast infections to digestive upset. Use this infusion daily to help prevent bacterial infections.

Ingredients:

1 cup fresh minced garlic

1 ½ cups extra-virgin olive oil

Instructions:

1. Place the garlic in a small glass jar and pour in the olive oil.
2. Cover the jar tightly with a lid and place in a sunny area.
3. Let the jar sit for 2 weeks, shaking twice a day to keep the garlic submerged.
4. After 2 weeks, strain the mixture through cheesecloth and discard the garlic.
5. Pour the oil back into the small jar and store in the refrigerator.
6. Add 1 teaspoon of the infusion to ½ cup of water and enjoy daily.

Sage Tincture for Sore Throat

Not only is sage known to help reduce fever and mucus production, but it is also a powerful herb for soothing a sore throat. This sage tincture is a simple way to reduce throat soreness – drink it in tea to enhance the soothing benefits.

Ingredients:

¼ cup dried sage, crushed

1 ¼ cups high-proof vodka

Glass pint jar

Instructions:

1. Pour the sage into the pint jar.
2. Add the vodka and stir until the herbs are fully saturated.
3. Screw the lid tightly onto the jar and place it in a cool, dark area.
4. Let the jar sit for 2 weeks, shaking it once daily.
5. Strain the mixture through a piece of cheesecloth, squeezing the liquid from the sage as much as possible.
6. Discard the solids and strain the liquid through a coffee filter.
7. Pour the liquid into small, dark-colored glass bottles.
8. To use, take ½ to 1 teaspoon of the tincture directly by mouth twice daily or add it to a cup of warm tea to enhance the benefits.

Turmeric Tea with Ginger

Both turmeric and ginger contain a powerful antioxidant called curcumin which helps to relieve muscle and joint pain. Both of these spices are known for their anti-inflammatory benefits which makes this tea a great herbal remedy for joint pain and arthritis.

Ingredients:

1 cup boiling water

¼ teaspoon ground turmeric

¼ teaspoon ground ginger

1 tablespoon raw honey

Instructions:

1. Combine the turmeric and ginger in a mug or tea cup.
2. Pour in the boiling water and stir gently.
3. Let the mixture steep for 5 minutes or so then stir in the honey and enjoy immediately.

Other Antibiotic Recipes

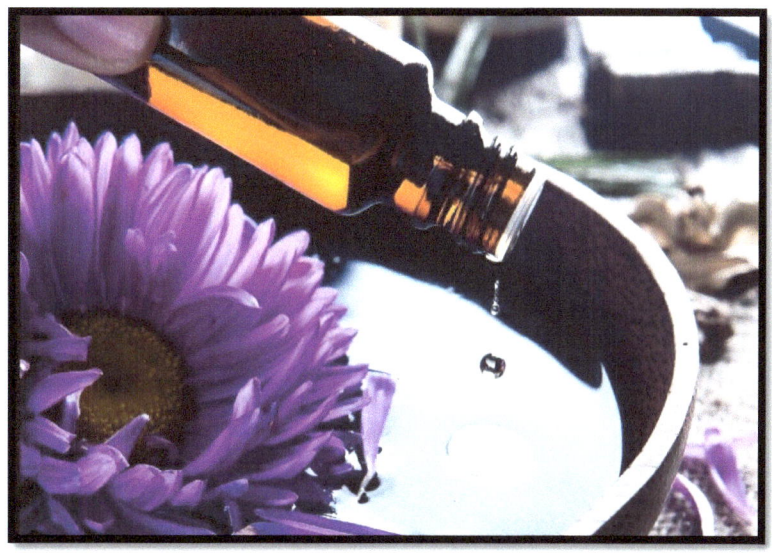

Recipes Included in this Section:

Honey Lemon Cough Syrup

Chapped Lip Balm

Oregano Oil Antibiotic Bath Salts

Soothing Peppermint Cough Syrup

Insect Bite Balm

Kid-Friendly Sore Throat Spray

Basil Oil Antibiotic Bath Salts

Natural Remedy for Earache

Kid-Friendly Cough Syrup

Toothache Clove Compress

Honey Lemon Cough Syrup

This honey lemon cough syrup is gentle and soothing, exactly what you need for a sore throat or cough. Feel free to add more or less honey according to your preference and consider swapping out the lemon zest for orange zest if you prefer a different flavor. This cough syrup is safe for children over the age of one

Ingredients:

1 cup water

1 cup raw honey

½ cup fresh lemon juice

1 tablespoon lemon zest

½ teaspoon ground ginger

Pinch ground clove

Instructions:

1. Whisk together the water, ginger, clove, and lemon zest in a small saucepan.
2. Bring the mixture to a boil over medium heat then reduce heat and simmer for 5 minutes.
3. Strain the mixture into a glass bowl and discard the solids.
4. Rinse the saucepan then add the honey and heat it over low heat.
5. Stir in the lemon juice and reserved liquid then simmer until it forms a thick syrup.
6. Pour the syrup into a glass jar and cover tightly with the lid – store in the refrigerator for up to 2 months.
7. To use, take 1 to 2 tablespoons every 4 hours for adults.

Note: For children aged 1 to 5, use ½ to 1 teaspoon every 2 hours. For children aged 5 to 12, use 1 to 2 teaspoons every 2 hours.

Chapped Lip Balm

This chapped lip balm is incredibly easy to prepare and it is very cost-effective – for the price of a single tube of commercial lip balm you can make half a dozen tubes using this recipe. Both coconut oil and beeswax help to soothe and moisturize chapped lips while myrrh essential oil adds its antibacterial power. Feel free to swap out other essential oils for the lavender to customize the fragrance of the lip balm.

Ingredients:

1 ounce coconut oil

½ ounce beeswax, grated

10 drops lavender essential oil

8 drops tea tree essential oil

5 drops myrrh essential oil

Instructions:

1. Combine the coconut oil and beeswax in a double boiler over low heat.
2. Heat the mixture until melted then stir to combine and remove from heat.
3. Stir in the essential oils until well combined.
4. Pour the balm into small containers and let set until firm.
5. Cover with the lids and store at room temperature.
6. Apply the balm to dry, chapped lips to soothe and heal.

Oregano Oil Antibiotic Bath Salts

All three of the essential oils used in this recipe for oregano oil antibiotic bath salts are known for their antibiotic properties. Oregano essential oil is a powerful anti-inflammatory and antiviral agent as well as an expectorant while basil and thyme essential oils can help soothe a sore throat. These antibiotic bath salts can help to soothe skin conditions while also loosening chest congestion.

Ingredients:

2 cups Himalayan pink salt, coarse

20 drops oregano essential oil

10 drops basil essential oil

10 drops thyme essential oil

Instructions:

1. Pour the Himalayan pink salt in to a large mixing bowl.
2. Add the essential oils and stir until well combined.
3. Transfer the mixture to a glass pint jar and cover tightly with the lid.
4. Store the salts in a cool, dry place until ready to use.
5. To use, add about ¾ cup of salts to a hot bath – hold the salts in your hand under running water to dissolve them.
6. Stir the bath gently by hand before getting in then soak for 30 minutes.

Soothing Peppermint Cough Syrup

This homemade peppermint cough syrup is made with a powerful combination of antibacterial and soothing ingredients. The whisky acts as an analgesic and the honey adds is antibacterial power while also coating and soothing a sore throat. Peppermint adds flavor to the syrup while also helping to relieve your cough.

Ingredients:

½ cup water

Juice from 1 lemon

¼ peppermint candy stick, crushed

¼ peppermint candy stick, whole

¼ cup Southern Comfort, whiskey

1 ½ cups raw honey

Glass jar

Instructions:

1. Whisk together the water and lemon juice in a small saucepan over medium heat.
2. Add the crushed peppermint stick and heat it until it is melted.
3. Remove from heat and cool for 5 minutes.
4. Stir in the whiskey and honey.
5. Place the remaining peppermint stick in a small glass jar.
6. Strain the liquid from the saucepan into the jar and discard the solids.
7. Let cool then cover tightly with the lid and store in a cool, dry place.
8. To use, take 1 to 2 tablespoons every 3 to 4 hours as needed.

Insect Bite Balm

This insect bite balm is made with a number of soothing and healing ingredients. Beeswax is a natural anti-inflammatory that helps to improve bacterial skin infections as well as soothing irritation and itching. Lavender essential oil adds a pleasing fragrance while tea tree oil moisturizes and heals. Basil essential oil adds its natural antibiotic benefits to the mix, helping to prevent infection and to speed healing.

Ingredients:

4 ounces coconut oil

2 ounces beeswax, grated

10 drops lavender essential oil

10 drops basil essential oil

8 drops tea tree essential oil

Instructions:

1. Combine the coconut oil and beeswax in a double boiler over low heat.
2. Heat the mixture until melted then stir to combine and remove from heat.
3. Stir in the essential oils until well combined.
4. Pour the balm into a clean metal container and let set until firm.
5. Cover with the lid and store at room temperature.
6. Apply the balm directly to the affected area to soothe and heal.

Kid-Friendly Sore Throat Spray

This sore throat spray is made with Echinacea, an herb known for its antibacterial properties and for its ability to soothe the symptoms of cold and flu. Not only is this throat spray effective, but it is also gentle enough to use on children.

Ingredients:

2/3 cups water

2/3 cups vegetable glycerin (food grade)

2 tablespoons dried Echinacea, crushed

2 tablespoons dried licorice root, crushed

½ tablespoon dried lemon zest

½ teaspoon dried Oregon grape root

Instructions:

1. Combine the water and vegetable glycerin in a glass jar.
2. Place the remaining ingredients in a coffee grinder and grind into powder.
3. Add the ground herbs to the jar and cover tightly with the lid.
4. Store in a cool, dry place for 2 weeks, shaking daily.
5. Strain the liquid through cheesecloth and discard the solids.
6. Pour the mixture into small spay bottles.
7. To use, shake well and spray on sore throat up to four times daily.

Basil Oil Antibiotic Bath Salts

Basil essential oil has been used to treat a variety of ailments including nausea, indigestion and constipation as well as various respiratory conditions. These basil oil antibiotic bath salts are a gentle way to soothe respiratory ailments while also helping to treat the symptoms of skin conditions like acne and various infections.

Ingredients:

2 cups Himalayan pink salt, coarse

20 drops basil essential oil

10 drops geranium essential oil

8 drops lavender essential oil

Instructions:

1. Pour the Himalayan pink salt in to a large mixing bowl.
2. Add the essential oils and stir until well combined.
3. Transfer the mixture to a glass pint jar and cover tightly with the lid.
4. Store the salts in a cool, dry place until ready to use.
5. To use, add about ¾ cup of salts to a hot bath – hold the salts in your hand under running water to dissolve them.
6. Stir the bath gently by hand before getting in then soak for 30 minutes.

Natural Remedy for Earache

Earaches are a painful condition that can be a nightmare for young children and their parents. Fortunately, it is easy to treat earaches naturally with a little garlic and mullein, an herb that is known for being gentle on children.

Ingredients:

1/2 cup dried mullein, crushed

¼ cup olive oil

1 tablespoon minced garlic

Instructions:

1. Combine the oil, garlic and mullein in a small saucepan.
2. Bring to a gentle boil then reduce heat and simmer for 2 hours.
3. Pour the mixture through a mesh strainer or cheesecloth and discard the solids.
4. Transfer the liquid to a small, dark glass bottle.
5. Use a dropper to apply a few drops of the liquid to the affected ear.

Kid-Friendly Cough Syrup

If you are looking for a cough syrup that is powerful enough to stop a cough but gentle enough for children, this is the perfect recipe. The honey coats and soothes the throat while adding its antibacterial power and the mullein gently treats the infection and relieves even the most stubborn of coughs.

Ingredients:

2 tablespoons dried mullein leaves, crushed

2 cups water

½ to 1 cup raw honey

Glass jar

Instructions:

1. Place the mullein in a small saucepan and cover with water.
2. Simmer the mixture on low heat for 15 minutes then strain through fine mesh or cheesecloth.
3. Pour the liquid back into the saucepan and simmer until reduced by half.
4. Remove from heat and whisk in the honey, stirring until it is dissolved.
5. Pour the syrup into a glass jar and cool to room temperature before covering tightly with the lid and storing in a cool, dry place.
6. To use for children aged 1 to 5, take ½ to 1 teaspoon every 2 hours. For children aged 5 to 12 take 1 to 2 teaspoons every 2 hours as needed.

Toothache Clove Compress

There are many things that can cause a toothache but, regardless the cause, relieving the pain can be tricky. Over-the-counter pain relievers can take a while to kick in and, in some cases, they do nothing to dull the pain. Your best option is to treat the pain directly at the source using a compress like this clove compress.

Ingredients:

Warm water

Epsom salt

1 teaspoon extra-virgin olive oil

6 drops clove essential oil

Cotton balls

Instructions:

1. Create a saltwater solution using the warm water and Epsom salts then gargle with it to clean out your mouth.
2. Stir together the olive oil and clove essential oil in a small bowl.
3. Dip a cotton ball in the oil mixture.
4. Press the cotton ball firmly against your sore tooth and hold it there for a few minutes to relieve pain.

Conclusion

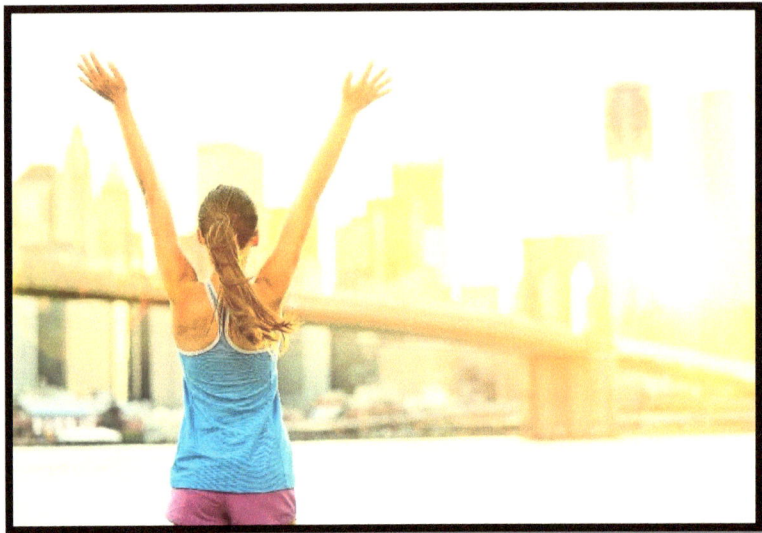

After reading this book you should have a firm understanding of what natural antibiotics are and how they can benefit you. While prescription antibiotics may sometimes do the trick, they often come with side effects and they may contribute to antibiotic resistance. If you want to tackle the problem head-on in an all-natural way, consider making your own antibiotic and antiviral remedies at home. The recipes in this book will help you to get started and, once you do, you will never go back.

I Need Your Help!

Please take a minute out of your busy schedule to leave a review.

Your review will let readers know what to expect and what you liked about this book. I am looking forward to reading your review.

Thank you so much for your feedback!

How to Submit a Review

To submit a review:

1. Make sure you are signed in.
2. Hover over **Your Account** in the upper right hand corner.
3. Click on **Your Orders**.
4. Click on **Digital Orders**.
5. Click **Write a customer review** in the Customer Reviews section.
6. Rate the item and write your review.
7. Click **Submit**.

How to submit a review from your Kindle device

Please follow the link below for instructions.

http://www.dummies.com/how-to/content/posting-an-amazon-book-review-from-your-kindle.html

www.ingramcontent.com/pod-product-compliance
Lightning Source LLC
Chambersburg PA
CBHW041515280526
45792CB00004B/1264